TANTRIC SEX

The 7 Nights To Awakening. A Step-By-Step Process To Unleash Your Sexual Energy, Touch Your Partner's Heart & Experience Ecstasy

ZOE LOXLEY

Table of Contents

INTRODUCTION... 3

The True Story Of Tantra - What Is And What Is Not ..7

Tantra & The Meaning Of Tantric Sex......................... 16

Tantrika: The Tantric Being That Is In Each Of Us....... 17

The 3 Golden Rules For Tantric Sex............................22

CHAPTER 1: Tantric Sex Concepts.. 27

The 4 Key Principles For Sexual Ecstasy..................... 30

The Orgasm In Tantric Sex..38

Pure Bliss: What Is The Valley Orgasm?..................... 42

How To Reach The Valley Orgasm?............................45

CHAPTER 2: Tantric Sex Techniques..................................... 49

The 10 Tantric Sex Positions..50

Tantric Positions With Chair............................... 56

Tantric Positions In Water.................................. 59

The Tantric Massage: What Is It & How To Do It........ 61

All The Benefits Of Tantric Massage............................63

Tantra Kundalini Massage... 64

CHAPTER 3: 7 Nights Of Tantra - Guide To Awakening......70

The First of 7 Nights...71

The Second of the 7 Nights.. 75

The Third of the 7 Nights...78

The Fourth of the 7 Nights... 80

The Fifth of the 7 Nights..,,82

The Sixth of the 7 Nights.. 85

The Seventh and Last Night of Tantric Sex.................90

CHAPTER 4: Tips To Enhance Your Intercourse.................. 93

Tantric Exercises.. 93

Tantric Techniques To Rebalance Energies.............. 100

Tantric Sexual intercourse: Useful Tips.................... 101

The Way Of Tao And The Way Of Tantra.................. 105

How To Help Reaching Orgasm................................. 107

CONCLUSION... 111

"Tantric sex is a unique experience, a philosophy of life, a doctrine that has little to do with the sexual positions of Kamasutra. It allows the body and mind to free themselves and experience intense, deep feelings of true bliss."

INTRODUCTION

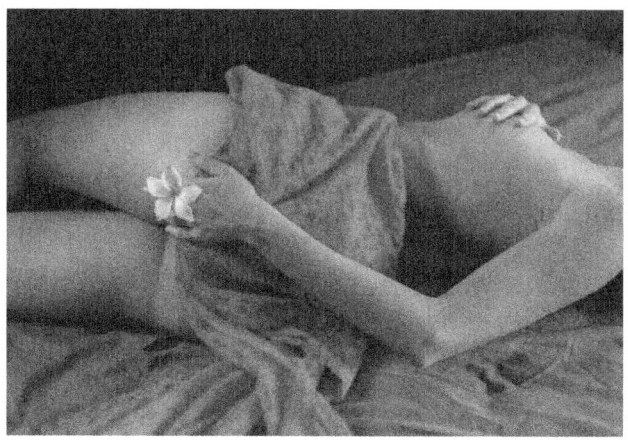

I t is a practice born in India around 400 B.C. and its aim has always been the knowledge and maturation of oneself. At that time, sexuality was in fact used to unite with the other and to ignite the spark of a person's nature. The word "tantra" is of Sanskrit origin, meaning principle, essence, technique and was used to indicate a series of spiritual teachings and esoteric traditions born in Indian religious cultures. As time went by, the term began to indicate that set of "sacred" sexual practices and rituals listed in Tantric literature that allow the body and mind to free themselves and experience almost supernatural sensations. In today's society, where sexuality is experienced more with the head than with the body, Tantric sex teaches the importance of slowness, attention, naturalness and complicity, all characteristics that deepen intimacy and increase passion, allowing you to communicate openly and authentically with your partner. Unlike traditional sex, in tantric sex it is essential to leave out the anxiety of orgasm, performance, result and you have to learn to enjoy eroticism in its totality, from sounds to breaths, up to movements.

Try to think about the typical sex, without romance: that's what you do quickly, with him often coming before her, few glances and many fixed thoughts. Will he see that I have cellulitis? Do I have it long enough for her? We are light years away from the concept of tantric sex, of slow and overwhelming spiritual and physical union that we all dream of as teenagers. You have surely heard of tantric sex thanks to some stars (Sting, anyone?), but few really know what they are talking about.

It's a real philosophy that tells us how to learn how to have sex for hours, how to prolong the pleasure to infinity and how to experience an extreme orgasm. Or not to feel it at all, discovering another level of pleasure where you don't need a sudden peak of sensations (incredible, but true!). If you are looking for a way to turn your sexual experiences as a couple into something supernatural, then we explain everything there is to know about tantra for two. And goodbye #frever to bad sex.

Tantric sex is recommended only for people who are particularly close because it is a more mental than physical practice that brings out all the problems and psychological motivations that are the basis of a relationship. At the same time, it is a practice that fights routine and allows you to create a deep, passionate connection, a real spiritual enlightenment. To deal with it in the best way, first of all, one should not be afraid to try something new. Only with an open mind and an open heart can you achieve total enjoyment. Then, you must decide to devote at least one hour a week to your sexuality, even when you are tired or stressed.

Tantric sex is in fact able to invigorate the body and make it stronger and more energetic. In addition, the atmosphere is very important to reach the peak of pleasure: the bedroom must be a magical space, a temple of love, a real feast of the senses. So it is good to decorate the bed with pillows, blankets, flowers, incense and even some fruit and some drinks. At this point, you will be able to relax, removing any blockages or tension that prevents the body to feel a deep and intense pleasure.

In tantric sex it is important to sit in front of your partner and meditate together with him, connecting your breath and your heart with that of the other. Although it may seem like a weird practice, once you try the positions of tantra the pleasure will turn into a real bliss. Tantric sex is a discipline open also to homosexuals, who can practice a sensual erotic massage to their partner. Such an intimate moment can make you rediscover your body and reach an extreme pleasure. Homosexuality in the East has never been considered a taboo and that's why such a passionate and intense sexual practice is open to any kind of gender.

The True Story Of Tantra - What Is And What Is Not

The original Tantra, also known as "Red" or "left hand" is linked to ancient matriarchal societies and has as its center the feminine energy. While the Tantra called "White" or "Right Hand", created later due to Muslim infiltration, derives from Indian patriarchal societies, as is the current Western one.

The difference between Red Tantra and White Tantra is radical. The second, White Tantra, is based on static and solitary meditations, while Red Tantra is a practice in which meditation is not only immobility and seriousness. In Red Tantra, meditation and sacredness are lived in every moment of existence, through deep listening and attention to what happens inside and outside of us. Meditation happens while dancing, working, hugging, eating, drinking, playing and talking.

There is a lot of confusion about what Tantra really is and especially a lot of targeted misinformation because of the persecution to which Original Tantra was subject. Tantra carries with it the burden of false clichés, such as free sex. Unlike other disciplines that have been less polluted, Tantra is for many a kind of Yoga practice; for others an orgiastic practice and for others a religion.

Summing up the only true Tantra is the one called Red. This does not mean that Tantra yoga, the white one and the one of the right hand, cannot be useful tools; but if you practice them you should at least know that you are not doing Tantra.

The Origins

According to the almost unanimous opinion of scholars, the archaic nature of the Red Tantra dates back to pre-Vedic cultures, to the very beginnings of Indian history, identifiable with the Harappei, Sindhu and other Dravidian populations who developed their Indus Valley civilization. According to some in the third millennium B.C. these populations were spread in a huge territory that went from Spain to the valley of the Ganges. Their precursors had settled in the Indus valley in Mehrgar starting from 7000 BC and their traces can be found until 5500 BC.

The Dravidian populations, therefore, appeared there around 6000-5000 B.C., had their apogee between 2300 and 1300 B.C. and disappeared, rather quickly, in a period of 100 years between 1900 and 1800 B.C. The reasons for their disappearance were attributed in the past to invasions of the Aryan population from the north. Today it tends to be attributed rather to a tectonic movement that raised the Aravali hills in the north of Rajastan, depriving the river that supported the Dravida civilization (the Ghaggar-Hakra) of most of its tributaries.

The Harappei population showed a strong interest in the arts and welfare. Theirs was a matriarchal society, the most important central monument of their city, was a large swimming pool; the element water was fundamental in their society and since then there was already a bath in every house. The woman was at the center of culture, centered on the mother goddess. The female figure dominated the sanctuaries and with open arms and legs, she offered herself for adoration.

The Harappei used to keep a large bed in the center of the most important room of the house and they practiced Tantra. Their religion was closely related to the body, well-being and sexuality.

It can be said that Red Tantra is the expression of all those practices that include sexuality. Red Tantra includes practices that also occur in groups, including contact and conveyance through the senses.

In the centuries following the birth of Tantra, in India, due to the Islamic invasions, the original Red Tantra was officially suppressed and forced to become an occult school. Thus was born the White Tantra, which had monastic aspects and was devoid of sexual intercourse; it was generally more tolerated but gradually lost its identity and merged with Yoga. Today we know it as Tantra Yoga, and it has completely lost its peculiarity of concrete approach to sexuality, typical of the original Tantra.

In practice, White Tantra is a Red Tantra but censored by all those practices that moralists could understand as disreputable. Today White Tantra, which is therefore a mystification of the original Tantra, is used in the West for commercial purposes. Almost all Tantra schools practice White Tantra and therefore do not really teach Tantra.

True Tantra is the Way of reconnecting with one's Self. It is the Way; the Way of the discovery of our genotypical sexual energies that are manifested through the knowledge and practice of the Tantra of Origin.

How it arrived in the West

At the same time with the sexual liberation of the 60s and 70s and the emancipation of women, some students and philosophers began to talk about Tantra and trying to make it a practice approachable even in the West, they made the rituals more agile and less blocking in the calculation of breathing and holding positions. Nowadays, emancipation allows women to get closer to the sexual world, although in Western society it is still believed that sex is more masculine than feminine and the cultural heritage does not allow women to focus on the fact that Tantra is a vehicle to achieve well-being and a higher spirituality.

In the West today Tantra aims to draw two maps, one that shows how to make the sexual experience spiritual and how to unite the earth to the sky, in a terrain where separation and judgment fade away and another map that brings us closer to the unknown sexual world (understood as unconditional love). A world, the Western world, where because of the Catholic religion and the like, there are no schools and traditions and everything is to be invented and experienced. In the West the sexual sphere is a world crushed for two millennia, by taboos and religions that often finds its only expression in private clubs or porn sites.

Tantra with all its erotic experiences is nothing more than a tool that opens physical, emotional and energetic internal spaces and opens to awareness.

Tantra is therefore only the Red Tantra. It is the EIA of liberation that opens to the true expression of one's Self and allows one to escape, both in the imaginary and in the real, from the dimension of the matrix in which sexual energy is mechanically channeled for improper purposes.

Sex and sexual energy are very different things.

The idea of sex is what settled in the imaginary during education, stories and commercial pornography; a program therefore, but so ingrained that individuals believe that it is precisely that pre-programmed way that sexual energy should be expressed. A program that is then gradually enhanced with repetitive experiences that are added together as memories.

The vital energy, or commonly known as sexual energy, is instead what is really the essence of man at its origin; it is what we carry in our genes, but because of the education received in the matrix, is then expressed in fact in an unnatural way.

The matrix has selected over time, with the help of religious morality, a sexual mode completely aimed at procreation ... so mechanical and centered on penetration and orgasm as a goal to be achieved, as if all the wonder of the contact between bodies should be enclosed in an act of a few minutes, between the two genitals. Many people believe they are free sexually because they make much of that mechanical sex, while in reality they are just more slaves; slaves to a trap in which true sexual energy is humiliated and crushed.

The true expression of sexual energy and every moment we love something, a flower, a sunset or a caress. And when that energy expresses itself free from the mechanisms inculcated in the mind, it becomes rite, celebration, connection of bodies, transcendence, healing energy, non-verbal communication, openness to trust between souls, breaking mechanical patterns, projection into the real and the imaginary of a world made of love. Because love cannot be sought... love is a fruit of the tree of freedom. It is therefore freedom that generates love and it is precisely by freeing oneself from the schemes that one encounters love.

Tantra & The Meaning Of Tantric Sex

The word *tantra* has a precise meaning: technique. It was born as a tantric philosophy of love that brings fullness and intimacy in a relationship through the use of specific sexual techniques. Tantra - also known as sex yoga - is above all love and a new way of seeing life. Tantra is sacred sex because man is the earthly manifestation of a God (Shiva) and woman of a Goddess (Shakti). During sex the woman - who is the active one of the two (you are warned) - must transfer her "cold energy" to the man who transforms it into "hot energy". The purpose of tantric practices is not to reach the couple's orgasm immediately, but to achieve sexual ecstasy for as long as desired. Cool to say, a little harder to get it.

Tantrika: The Tantric Being That Is In Each Of Us

It seems that tantrika, historically, although Tantra had not identified the other matrix, the living one, is a representation adherent to that of the Essence of the Original Free Man.

The Tantra of Origin provides nothing but elementary conditioning, morality and prohibitions (i.e. the grid of the individual matrix-slave) from one's own mind, in order to bring out the Self. The following points should therefore be understood, exclusively, in what remains after eliminating this matrix from one's mind, nothing else. Thus, the void created by the cleansing of the antimatrix becomes the emptiness-full.

The tantrika does not live nor does the couple, together with the materialism of the superfluous, as the primary factor of the matrix-slave that disconnects the individual from unconditional universal love, to bring him into the conditioned one, in which the double-matrix operates. He is therefore aware that in "normal" life love does not exist, because calling love the conditional Love is only a euphemism.

1) FREEDOM FROM EXPECTATIONS:

Meaning lack of a foreshadowing of what has to happen and therefore freedom from disappointment when what you wanted does not come true. So tantrika has its own center of gravity that is not dependent on the outside and is not affected by the failure of something or its transformation into something else. Ability then to let go without dwelling on the negative and allow it to alter the soul. The tantrika lives in the HERE AND NOW.

2) FREEDOM FROM SENTIMENTALITY:

Meaning the absence of slipping into pietism and the condescension of religiosity. The tantric way requires a centrality and an ability to observe clearly if one cheats with oneself.

3) FREEDOM FROM THE CONCEPT OF SIN:

Meaning not taking into account the judgment of others because on tantrika have not taken into account the appreciation of the society in which he lives (whether positive or negative appreciation) and therefore much less the moral concepts.

4) FREEDOM FROM FEAR:

understood as the ability 'to overcome both physical and psychological fears that do not advance us on our inner journey and that can become disabling and restrictive for ourselves.

5) FREEDOM FROM DISGUST:

understood as the possibility not to be bound in practice and life by insuperable sensations that prevent us from having an experience, experience being a fundamental aspect of tantric knowledge.

6) FREEDOM FROM THE FAMILY:

Conceived as freedom from family ties and beliefs and from the wrapping mechanisms of the family of origin and ultimately in the ability to distance themselves from the familiar clichés that tend to control and manipulate the other.

7) FREEDOM OF ORIGIN:

Meaning freedom and the possibility of being above all differences in race, skin color, origin and origin. The one who wants to produce the fire does not care which tree the wood he finds belongs to.

8) FREEDOM TO THE INTERDICTIONS:

Understanding as moral constraints or social conformism and therefore freeing the will 'from all laws and ability' to distance themselves from them so as to break the chains of the schemes.

9) FREEDOM FROM THE COUPLE AND MONOGAMY:

Meaning freedom to express the genotype, since monogamy and the couple are not in the nature of man who, like 97% of mammals, has oxytocinic mechanisms that make him genotypically polygamous.

"Free souls vibrate and create the melodies of the cosmos. Sometimes their music touches each other, in moments of symphonies that attract dancing, unique pearls of a universe that plays with forms". Cit. Almalibre Rebelde

10) FREEDOM FROM RELIGIOUS AND POLITICAL SLAVE-MATRIX:

Understood as freedom to be in the genotypical human space-time variant of the here and now; a dimension in which neither dogmas nor social can exist.

11) FREEDOM TO LIVE IN THE DIMENSION OF UNCONDITIONAL UNIVERSAL LOVE.

It is understood as the awareness that love is not a point of arrival and that it cannot be searched for, because this dimension, that of unconditional universal love, is revealed after the liberation of the self, from the matrix-slaughterer's hood. Unconditional universal love is therefore a dimension fruit of self liberation.

The 3 Golden Rules For Tantric Sex

What are the rules to make the best tantric sex and enjoy its full benefits? First of all, we must say that this is recommended only to people who are already united by a particular relationship. It is not good, therefore, for one-time relationships, but it is much better to put it in a couple context. The affinities will be greater, precisely because it serves to improve all the problems that are the basis of a relationship.

Another rule to enjoy tantric sex is not to be in a hurry. This type of sexuality is in fact, very different from what we all know that, lately, is rather dominated by the cold. Here you can dedicate yourself to your sexuality calmly. This is the only way to achieve total enjoyment. Tantric sex allows you to invigorate the body and make it stronger and more energetic. The atmosphere is very important to carry it out. Yes, therefore, to pillows, special lights, drinks and flowers, to make the environment more welcoming. In fact, it is necessary to relax completely in order to carry it out and to have an intense and lasting pleasure.

First, two people sit opposite each other. You go to connect your breath with the other person first. It sounds like a strange practice but in reality, once you try it, it can really turn into something pleasant. Tantric sex is not something related only to heterosexuality. It is a discipline that also opens to homosexuality and, therefore, even people of the same sex can practice sensual erotic massages to their partner.

It is also true in fact, that homosexuality in the East has never been a taboo, contrary to what often happens in the West. There are many VIPs who have claimed to perform tantric sex. Among them stands out the singer Sting who, years ago, revealed that through this practice, he manages to make sex last for several hours, even continuously.

First of all it is necessary to know your body well, before approaching this philosophy of oriental origin. This happens in the acquisition of awareness of our muscles, but also bones and nerves. Not only about pleasure centers, but about the whole body. Awareness then, must be extended to thoughts and actions. One must pay attention and train concentration. Another suggestion comes from movements, which can be done either alone or in pairs.

There are in fact, movements that help in the synchronization of gestures. You should not decide a priori the positions of tantric sex, because otherwise it would lose all its meaning.

Tantra is in fact, something sacred and a freedom of movement. Through a reciprocal massage we can help in the process of knowledge: a massage oil, therefore, can be the only accessory that can serve in tantric sex. Thanks to it you can also get the so-called valley orgasm. What does it consist of? It is a sense of bliss that comes from the degree of intimacy achieved with the partner and not through the mere sexual act.

Since tantra is mutual pleasure, there should be no inhibitions. In this regard, you can also use your voice, if you want. Nothing to do with dirty talking. You talk with whispers, you let your voice flow, you let yourself go in sounds that can be pleasant. Finally, you have to consider that a fundamental role is played by breathing. This should be synchronized as much as possible, in the most natural way. In this way, for example through an embrace, you can exactly perceive your partner's movement and breath and adjust accordingly.

Tantra is something that has nothing to do with selfishness and offers no room for absence. This is all we need to know about the oriental sexual practice of tantric sex, which we have seen have millennial origins. In the West there are some variants of tantric sex, although they are not exactly identical. The real tantra belongs to the East and is no longer even what is practiced today, but what was once done.

CHAPTER 1: TANTRIC SEX CONCEPTS

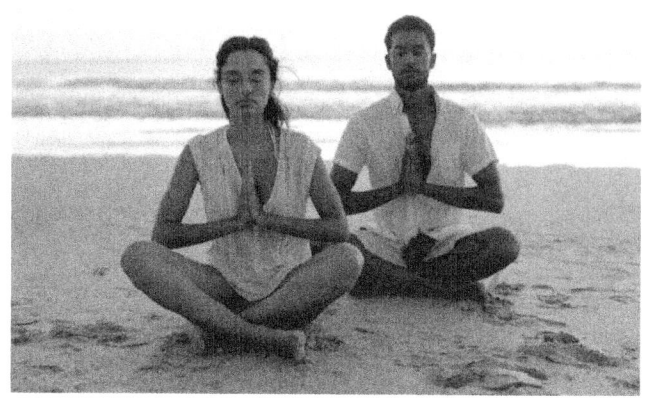

Many people wonder if tantric sex really works. To make it an intensely erotic moment within the couple you need to follow a series of "tricks". First of all it is necessary to focus on your body and the rhythm of movement, so as to promote the circulation of energy. Voice emissions should not be blocked or inhibited for any reason. In tantric sex you should feel free to express

100% of your pleasure. Finally, breathing deeply also helps to achieve pleasure.

To improve results, there are exercises to be performed together with your partner to improve the whole sphere of sexual affectivity. For example, you can learn to breathe the right way using your diaphragm. You have to breathe in counting to six, hold your breath for another six seconds and exhale for another six. In addition, women must understand where the perineal area is, it can be used to stimulate orgasm only with the pelvic muscles, without any sudden movement. The key to making tantric sex work is to listen to your body, reviewing its different parts and related sensations.

It starts from the first attitude to put into practice or listening: you have to feel and become aware of every inch of your body, understand what gives you pleasure and then get in touch with your emotions at an intimate level never experienced before. You have to get rid of all the stress of everyday life but also of all those limitations that prevent you from letting go, such as low self-esteem and dislike on a physical level. It can help to create before making love a relaxing situation, with candles, soft lights, a massage with scented oil, in short, what you like best.

There are also some tantric exercises to learn to go at the same pace as your partner, so as not to think about sex as a sports performance all projected on the final orgasm. If you surrender to your feelings you can be able to enjoy every single moment without reaching the orgasmic peak (the so-called *valley orgasm*).

Fundamental is also the use of the voice, which frees the chest and the pelvis: don't keep the sounds inside you, let them out because they allow you to open your mind.

But the most important aspect of tantra is the relationship between breathing and sexuality: to make love well, in short, you must also learn to breathe well, deeply, to be able to amplify every feeling.

The 4 Key Principles For Sexual Ecstasy

According to tantra there are 4 keys to overcome the psychophysical limits of pleasure, that are:

- Attention - body awarness,
- movement and rhythm,
- the sound,
- the breath.

It is not about looking for the right partner or situation, but about looking inside yourself and expanding your sexual energy. By opening one door at a time we can enrich our emotional and sexual life.

But how do we do it? Our body is naturally endowed with the 4 keys to pleasure: you just have to learn how to make them turn the right way, to open access to a new erotic dimension.

The attention or body awareness

The first key to pleasure is attention, understood as body awareness. Using this key means learning to listen to your body, first separately, then together with your partner. In what way?

For example, with this exercise, divided into three moments.

First of all, close your eyes, put on relaxing music and focus on the various parts of the body: feet, legs, pelvis, neck...". Those who have difficulty can make small movements to make contact. Then, try to understand how all the parts of your body are, to feel them.

The second part of the exercise is about emotionality: what emotions, what feelings, what climate is inside me? Where do I feel that feeling or this emotion? What is there, in that point?".

Finally, conclude the exercise by composing some mental visualizations that start from this thought: "if I was on a train and I saw my thoughts passing, what would they be and what would they say about me?

During the sexual intercourse we have to pay attention to our body, to the contact area of our physicality with each other, and to the resulting body sensation. Stay in that feeling, do not follow the thoughts, especially those that begin with "duty" (e.g. I should be more excited, etc.). Rather, ask yourself this question: "what do I feel in my body when I make love?"".

Movement and rhythm

The second key to pleasure is represented by movement and rhythm, and this is what tantra says allows the circle of energy. That is why it is important to move together with your partner, in order to unlock them, especially at the level of the pelvis.

To harmonize your rhythm with that of your partner, you can try cycling exercise: sit against your seat, hold your hands and start cycling. The first step is to learn to move together; then you need to synchronize in order to find a shared rhythm. See how long it takes you to find it, who is leading, who is slowing down, who is struggling to keep up. Finally, try some variations on the theme: while pedaling, make some movements (like arching your back), help you find the rhythm and then vary the pattern. During the intercourse everyone should be able to move in total freedom.

During the exercise, try to put body jazz music in the background, to learn how to move even by yourself, and so to loosen the body first the neck, then the shoulders, progressively descending and prepare it to follow all forms of pleasure.

The sound

The third key to pleasure is the voice, with all its vibrations and sound. The vocal emissions and sounds coming out of the throat, in fact, free the mind, unlock the chest and the belly (pelvis), and therefore the pleasure. Do not hold them back (it is not mandatory to "shout"), let them flow into the body and then out of the throat, naturally: it is self-exciting, and helps to put sexual energies into circulation.

Breathing

The fourth key to pleasure is breathing, which according to tantra, can also be the most devious way to inhibit pleasure and excitement, because if the breath is short or shallow, we do not oxygenate our body well: it is like starting in fourth gear, but with the handbrake pulled.

Learning to breathe well, deeply, therefore, is fundamental, for example with this simple exercise:

The breath must be soft and circular. As you breathe in, count to 6, hold for another 6 and release, always counting up to 6, because the phases of breathing must be symmetrical. If you practice in this way, you begin to change not only your breathing, but also the way you perceive your body. When you are in a couple, then, as for the movements, it is important to synchronize the breath with that of the partner, because this allows all the energy to circulate and amplify the sensations. And also the emotions: according to the oriental philosophy, by taking 3 deep breaths when you embrace a person you love very much, you double your happiness.

Some men might be a bit skeptical to try tantric sex, which proposes a different approach to sexuality from the "western" one. How to convince him? Instead of many speeches, a playful mode that can give immediate pleasure can be useful. For example, starting with a sensual massage, taking time to explore sensoriality. And then, lead him into this new erotic dimension, taking on the role of geisha: be sure that he will rely on your guidance.

To summarize...

Tantra and its techniques are not easy, but neither are impossible. Be careful: tantric practices are for very close couples. They will prove to be an epic fail if they lack great confidence, feeling and desire at the top. Ready to give it a try? There is no need to buy a guide to tantric sex, just start getting involved with the four basic tantric exercises:

- **Live the present moment and be aware of your body:** listen to your and her body, listen to your breathing, look intensely into each other's eyes, love every detail of each other. There is no space to think about what you have to do next, what commitments you have to fix, what problems at work you have, what physical defects your partner might see. During tantric love you love every detail of yourself and your partner. No mental limit, no physical limit, no prejudice. Kiss each other, touch each other, observe each other all the time in the relationship.

- **Rhythm and movement are fundamental:** they put energy into circulation and must be done in harmony. You move together, at the same speed, possibly slowly and deeply, especially at the pelvis level. No rush into penetration, please. It must be almost a dance.

- Tantra breathing is a must: how to prolong the pleasure if not by controlling the breath? The more relaxed and soft it is, the more it oxygenates the erogenous zones. The top would be to synchronize your breath with that of your partner: try to inhale counting to six, hold your breath for six seconds and exhale for another six.

- Prolonged coitus: the sensations are so deep that you will naturally postpone your orgasm. It won't have to be your goal, you won't have to chase it, but neither will you have to hold it if you feel it exploding. He doesn't even need a full erection: it is enough that the penis remains inside you to stimulate it with the contraction of the pelvic muscles and continue to feel a super pleasure. It's called valley orgasm and it comes from listening to the sensations: the warmth, the softness of the skin, the scent, the features of your partner and so on.

The Orgasm In Tantric Sex

That orgasm is the crowning achievement of sexual intercourse is something we take for granted. On the contrary, when it is not achieved (constantly), perplexities, crises and finally couple problems begin. Yes, because in Western society, sex has a linear approach: from courtship to the sexual act, which ends with orgasm, possibly both. But not for everyone is so. In Tantric sex, for example, this view fades.

Tantra is a set of doctrines based on the principle of transgression. The transgression was primarily that of the order based on purity.

But Tantrism has always had an objective that goes beyond the simple violation of the rules. Simplifying a lot, one could say that in Tantrism the person questions his own person as he has always understood it. The goal is an overcoming of the subjectivity of the individual, his values and his identity. This process in the Tantric vision leads man in a dimension where he comes into contact with his true self and therefore with the divine dimension.

In the tantric vision of sex, pleasure is not the point of arrival, as some believe. Often, in fact, we hear about intense orgasms and legendary performances. But the matter is much more complex because even sex becomes a means. It is part of a systematic project to get in touch, through pleasure, with one's deep self.

Among the characteristics of tantric sex, as far as men are concerned, there is the practice of semen retention. Orgasm, as we understand it in the West, does not actually happen. This practice produces an accumulation of energy that is not released through ejaculation. In short, man manages to control a process that in the eyes of many is pure abandonment of control. The accumulated energy, often called kundalini, goes up towards the upper part of the body. In this way you reach an ecstatic state that goes far beyond simple physical pleasure.

This state can only be reached thanks to a very complex path that is difficult to achieve in the West. It is not a path for everyone. It requires a solid yogic training, ability to control emotions, ascetic practice and spiritual maturity. It is also necessary to pass through the experience of emptiness, a test not suitable for everyone, which involves advanced meditative skills.

Tantrism is for many people synonymous with freedom, deriving from the abandonment of the rules; it is no coincidence that it began to fascinate the West in '68, a period of great claims in this sense. However, it has often been mystified, made a sort of pass for epic sexual experience.

Yes, because we often think we can use superficially practices from other cultures, as if they were shortcuts for the purposes we set out for (and in fact in the West tantra has also known a light version known as neotantra). It is not a test to do with tantric sex, which is a dangerous operation. It is an extreme way reserved for a few; if you are not ready, it is easy to be a victim. Not everyone, in fact, is prepared to make contact with their own depths and manage the disruptive force of some emotions. "Tantric sex is reserved for the hero, that is to say, the one who is able to bear the liberation of energy that comes from it.

Although not within everyone's reach, this practice retains a remarkable charm, as well as an extremely equal view of the relationship. The ideal tantric union presupposes an equality between man and woman. Both must be aware of the mystical purpose of sexual practice. And both see themselves as divinities: they are the mirror of a divine image of each other. In sexual intercourse they "die", they dissolve, one into the other; as the Persian mystics write, what remains at the end of the union between lover and beloved is only Love.

Pure Bliss: What Is The Valley Orgasm?

Have you ever heard of valley orgasm? At first glance, this expression suggests that it is a dichotomous concept with another: where there is a valley there is also a mountain. And indeed it is so: "mountain orgasm" and "valley orgasm" are in fact concepts related to tantric sex, so let's talk about the spiritual side of sex and sexuality. There is a lot of talk about tantric sex - and many people call it an urban legend, a myth - but tantra is real, even if you need to deepen the discipline - there are also special seminars - and what we are going to tell you is for information purposes only.

One of the ways in which orgasm is usually indicated is "climax", i.e. peak. But that climax is actually the so-called mountain orgasm.

To understand, let's go behind the figurative image: a mountain, drawn as a fixed stereotype, is a large inverted V, in which there is an ascent, a vertex and a descent. In this similarity, the ascent is represented by all those actions that are carried out when having sex - from foreplay, to penetration, to the change of position, and so on. When you get to the top of the mountain, you feel the orgasm of the mountain, but the descent is sweet and pleasant, not fast and immediate. The mountain orgasm does not disappear immediately, but if "cultivated" in the right way, it can allow you to reach the valley orgasm.

Tantric sex can lead to the so-called valley orgasm. It may sound absurd but to achieve it you have to do absolutely nothing. Usually when making love you feel anxiety and tension because the goal is to make a good impression. In this practice of Indian origin, however, you do not have to worry about anything, it is not even necessary that the penis is erect. The intimate contact alone is enough. You need to have the muscles of the body relaxed and, at most, stimulate the male penis by contracting the pelvic muscles. The movements must be very slow and intense. Valley orgasm is a pleasure that comes from listening to simple sensations such as perfume, warmth, softness of the skin, partner's features, it is something that can only be achieved when anxiety, stress and effort are completely forgotten. The result, however, will be particularly intense, almost a form of bliss.

In the article The Art of Loving on Osho's website we read an invitation not to break away after having reached both orgasm: if you don't break away you can reach the valley orgasm, a state of deep well-being and closeness, love and meditation that somehow interpenetrate as the two bodies have interpenetrating just before. But it is possible only through silent observation, just before returning to normal, to the state that precedes coitus. Afterwards there can also be moments of pampering, indeed they are very important, almost essential, perhaps through massages with oils, good music and a little scented candles.

How To Reach The Valley Orgasm?

To reach orgasm in the valley... nothing must be done. Yes, it may seem absurd to you, but in fact all the action has taken place before and the valley orgasm is precisely the speculative and meditative phase of the relationship.

Attention, however: this does not mean that immediately after the relationship you have to put on your clothes or go to sleep, this is precisely what the tantra advises you to avoid. Sex is a sacred moment and must be treated as such. So let's go through the stages of the relationship to better understand how to behave and to make the most of sex as an experience that combines body and soul.

You are in bed - or wherever you like - with your partner or partner. There are the preliminaries and then the actual relationship that may or may not include penetration. The relationship culminates in the upstream orgasm - when and if it arrives - after which you take your time. Remaining close, embraced, in contemplation. The ideal is to reach the climax together, but it is something that can come about through deep mutual knowledge and practice - sometimes even of a sentimental nature, not just distinctly sexual. So after the climax you stay still, enjoy the moment, without being caught unprepared by what is usually called the refractory period and which leads to post-coital sleepiness.

And after that? You may be pervaded by a feeling of well-being that lasts for hours. Because your soul - as well as of course your body - has found fulfillment in what happened between the sheets.

Tantric sex obviously can't be improvised, it requires a physical but above all mental preparation, not doing anything of what one is usually led to do arouses many perplexities in Western culture. Those who practice tantric love define this experience as "cosmic" or "divine", it is a flow of energies that flow from the bodies, away from thoughts, from the pursuit of pleasure and the stress that comes with it. It is no coincidence that Western society has to deal with performance anxieties of all kinds and types, from erection problems to the female ones of never reaching orgasm.

Speaking in technical terms the tantric one is defined "Valley Orgasm" precisely because there is no need to reach the climax of pleasure, this feeling of "arrive - not arrive" is already very pleasant and deep, so that orgasm is really a surplus, an optional.

As we were saying, psychological preparation is essential, one cannot approach tantra if one does not deeply believe in making love as something beyond orgasm, penetration, it is something spiritual and intense that disorientates and leaves one almost interdicted.

CHAPTER 2: TANTRIC SEX TECHNIQUES

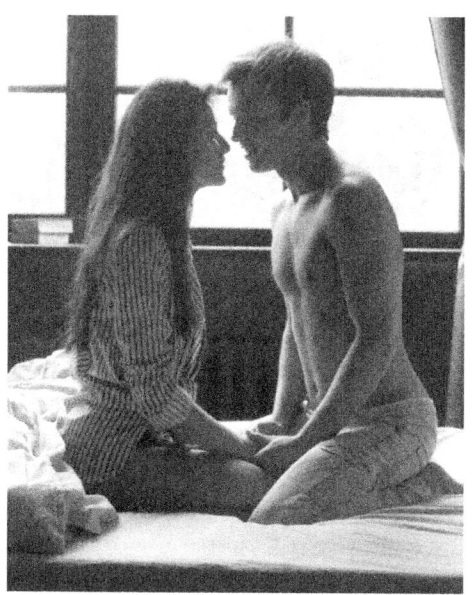

antric sex aims at the full sharing of emotions, sensations, both physical and mental. It unhinges the voracity typical of modern sexuality, understood as a pure vehicle of carnal pleasure, aimed at achieving a pleasant orgasm. Calmness, slowness and sharing are the basis, instead, of this doctrine that aims, as an objective, the improvement of sexuality, always, as clarified, passing from awareness and sharing of feelings and emotions.

The tantra practices focus, in fact, on the visual attention of the lovers, on tactile sensations, passing through the symbiosis of breath. Movement and rhythm, especially in the part of the pelvis, are the key words of tantric sex, these are what put in circulation a lot of energy, more than what we think we hide inside us, allowing us to unlock them, renewing the pleasure of the senses and the inner one. Tantric sex aims to allow those who practice it to better know both their body and that of their partner, encouraging the harmony of the couple.

The 10 Tantric Sex Positions

Taking new positions can help renew the passion. Before reviewing the best positions of tantric sex, it is necessary to follow some very specific preliminaries in order to achieve full physical and mental satisfaction.

In this regard, partners during tantric love must find themselves in a condition of complete relaxation. They must observe and contemplate themselves. Only when this balance will be achieved, only when the outpouring of glances and breaths will be maximum, then and only then you can proceed. Tantra positions can help you get started the right way. These 4 main positions look like yoga positions for couples and will make you feel fused together:

- **Lotus position:** the most famous one, made a cult by Sting himself (who told the press that he could have tantric sex for more than 7 hours in a row. Not bad!). Him sitting, her sitting on his thighs wrapping him with her own legs and holding him in a hug while moving rhythmically. Looking into his eyes it's the key.
- **Variant of the lotus position:** sitting facing each other, legs intertwined to merge into the penetration.

- **Position of the hot chair:** him sitting on the chair and leaning against the backrest, her sitting on him with her legs leaning against his shoulders.

- **Variant of the position of the hot chair:** both kneeling, he behind her pushing from behind while she makes circular movements with her pelvis. Super hot.

Lotus Position

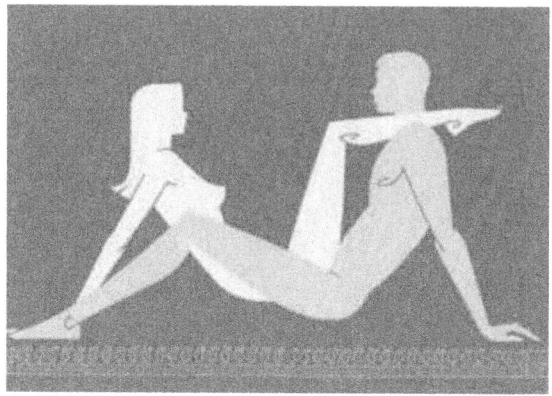

Perhaps the best known among the tantric sexual positions to be exploited in bed is that lotus flower where the man stands cross-legged with the woman on top of him, crossing his thighs behind his partner's back to wrap him and look him intensely in the eyes.

Lotus Variant

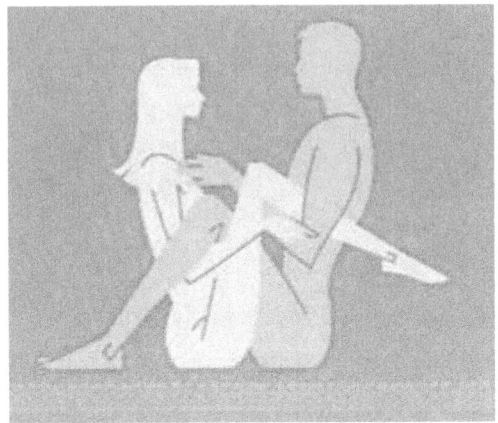

This basic tantric position can have several variations, such as the one where man and woman are sitting opposite each other and the legs intertwine almost as if to create a unique being perfectly fused together.

Ground Position

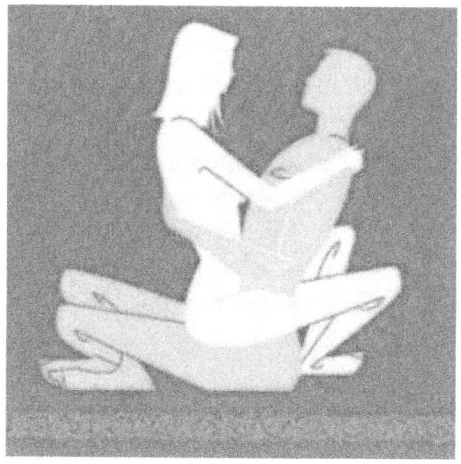

The typical position with him sitting and her on top of him is great to try even lying on the floor, or with pillows to make the intercourse more comfortable.

Tantric Positions With Chair

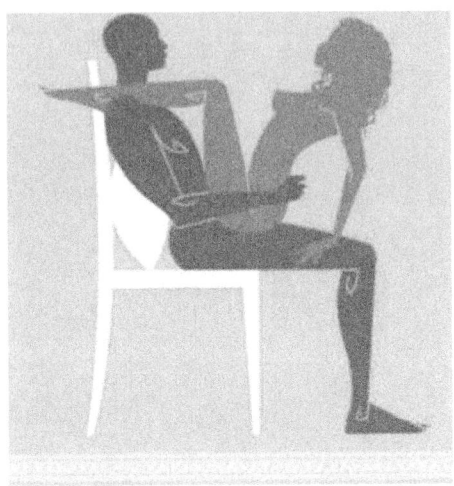

The most acrobatic lovers, who want to try new tantric positions, can also achieve pleasure with the help of a chair, where the seated man can welcome the woman who puts her legs over her partner's shoulders.

Crouching

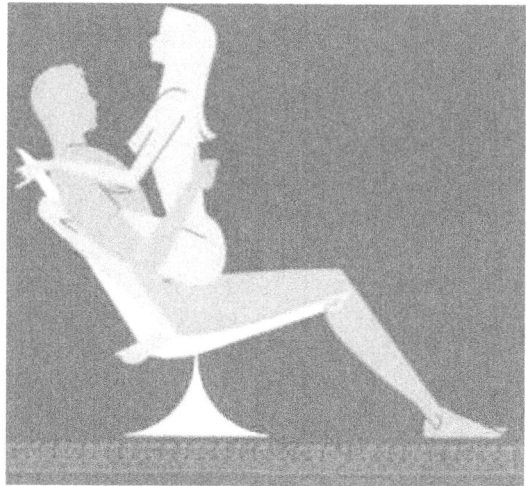

Among the best tantric sexual positions to try with a chair is also the one in which the woman is squatting over the man resting her feet on the edge.

The Bomb

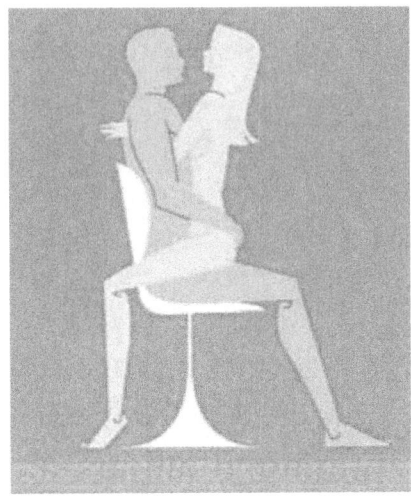

The tantric position of the bomb involves the man sitting on a chair and the woman on top of him, without touching the ground with her feet.

Tantric Positions In Water

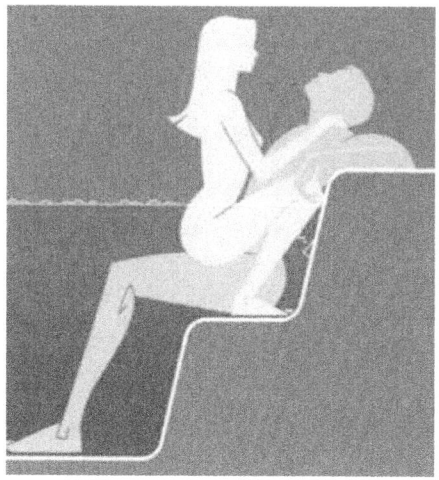

Tantra can also be safely put into practice in water, for example on a swimming pool, with the man sitting on the ladder and the woman crouched over him.

Tantric Position In Bathtub

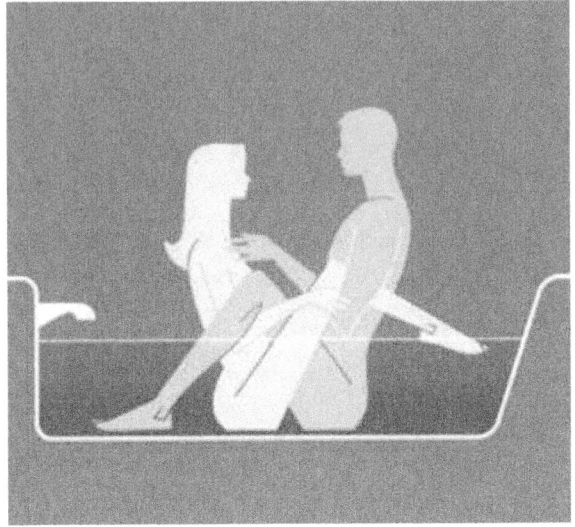

If you have a bathtub at home, you can try the classic tantric sexual position with hot water as an additional sexy and relaxing ingredient.

Tantric sex is the key to open the doors of pleasure, release sexual energy, allowing you to experience special sensations while experiencing very long intercourse times. This discipline of oriental origins changes the approach to sex, which is declined as a tool to achieve harmony of the senses, harmony of the couple, inner and outer balance, all passing from a unique and extremely captivating sensory experience.

The Tantric Massage: What Is It & How To Do It

Tantric massage is an ancient Indian practice that, through light and circular touches, stimulates the knowledge of oneself, of the other and leads to a state of well-being that is both union and liberation: let's see all the advantages.

Through tantric masasggio and stimulation of certain energy points of the body, the person who receives it experiences a great sensory pleasure and at the same time an improvement in self-perception and awareness. It is a good massage for those who want to increase and increase the knowledge and harmony of the couple. Tantric massage is based on ancient Indian teachings, which in turn date back to texts of pre-vedic cultures, the origin of which is still quite mysterious and controversial. The ancient population of the Harappa, for example, who occupied some parts of India thousands of years ago, gave great importance to the energy generated by tantra, in particular the female figure and its element, water; in the center of their houses there was a large swimming pool and a room with a large bed on which to practice tantric massage.

How To Do The Tantric Massage

The tantric massage is structured in three phases.

> In the first phase we focus on meditation and meditation, creating in a suitable and intimate place, such as the bedroom, a cozy environment, with soft

lighting, incense, practicing breathing exercises and reciting mantras.

> The second phase is focused on slow, circular and light massages on face and body, from legs to arms, passing through the pelvic area, back, neck and head, with gentle touches along the vital energy channels, chakras and nadi. A warm and delicate vector oil, such as coconut oil, is used.

> The last phase is relaxation: sipping a warm herbal tea you share the experience with those who have practiced it, verbalizing what you have experienced. Advantages of tantric massage.

All The Benefits Of Tantric Massage

Thanks to this type of message, those who receive it - but also those who offer it - will enjoy advantages and benefits, including a new experience of sexuality, not limited in space and time, but perceived as omnipresent energy to be channeled into every cell of the body. In this way, anxiety, stress concerns are dissolved, along with other tensions.

Far from being a sexual practice, tantric massage acts on the genitals by dissolving blockages and going to relax the first chakra, using Tantra lingam techniques for men and Tantra yoni for women. There is also the technique of Tantra Kundalini massage. Personal growth and sensory experience aimed at well-being go hand in hand in tantric massage, a practice that is especially aimed at rediscovering the sacredness of the body as an element and physical envelope of the soul.

Tantra Kundalini Massage

This is probably one of the most curious, fascinating and sensual forms of tantra massage: we are talking about the Kundalini technique, which ideally represents a snake, which in turn symbolizes the primordial energies that reside in each of us, to be precise at the first chakra. The snake is the metaphor of transformation, in reference to its peculiarity of losing and rebuilding the skin regularly, and the transformation is associated with well-being in physical and spiritual terms as well as enlightenment (remember that the tantra philosophy aims at the elevation of the individual).

The Kundalini tantric massage, in particular, awakens the primordial energy of the first chakra - located in the perineal area - the starting point for a tantra massage that also involves the genital areas, without excluding any part of the body, until reaching the seventh chakra, the top of the neck.

During the Kundalini tantra massage the chakras should be progressively purified, so that the Kundalini - i.e. primordial energy - can get the upper hand by breaking down obstacles such as attachment to physical and material pleasure (this is linked to sexual intercourse seen as an act of donation not necessarily aimed at orgasm), as well as to our ego. At the moment of Kundalini's awakening, in the recipient of this specific tantra massage, thanks to the harmonious and enveloping movements with which it is massaged, the entire body will experience a feeling of complete well-being and total pleasure.

The effectiveness of the massage can be achieved thanks to very prolonged manipulations (even two hours) performed by an experienced operator: do not try this massage without mastering the technique perfectly. The purpose of the massage is to promote relaxation of the muscles adjacent to the spine, to prepare the central channel (sushumua) to welcome the upward flow of kundalini energy. Once the back, shoulders and neck are open, the lower back, including legs, feet and buttocks, must be massaged vigorously to release tension in the lower extremities to facilitate kundalini upward flow.

With the back of the body relaxed, the lower pelvic area is prepared to be relaxed and opened through a circular deep massage into the sacral and pelvic area. In this way the main natii or astral canal is purified so that the kundalini currents can flow and join the Vishnu. The direction is always from bottom to top. For this reason, the work on the body starts at the bottom. The chakra centers are opened and balanced in order, from the bottom, then from the muladhara chakra, to the other, through the other chakra centers to the sahasrara. This opening serves to prepare the body for further releases and movements of kundalini energy.

When the lower pelvic cavity begins to open thanks to deep massage, the upper chakra siri must be prepared with gentle touches along the thorn in the direction of the neck. The highest chakra, ajna, and the Sahasrara area at the top of the head, are prepared for the opening through an energetic balance obtained without contact with the body. The opening of the subsequent chakras will create a passage that will allow the kundalini to radiate upwards. This first part of the massage, in which the recipient is lying face down, is preparatory to the second part, in which he will be lying on his back.

Once the chakra centers are activated, the kundalini energy contained in the muldhara chakra, placed at the base of the column, is gently released. The kundalini energy is often called "snake energy" because it lies inert, coiled at the base of the vertebral axis; it is static and sealed at the root of the spine, just beyond the tip of the sacrum. Releasing this energy creates two forces, one centripetal (Shakti) and the other centrifugal (Shiva). Shakti is directed upward to the highest chakras, to complete a union with Shiva. whose original source, according to Tantra, is the sun. It is thanks to the union of these two forces that harmony and balance are achieved, according to ancient Tantric beliefs.

Often the first experience of releasing kundalini energy is disappointing: the energy hardly rises above the first or second chakra. However, after a number of sessions that varies from subject to subject, the release of "awakened" kundalini energy takes place: those who have experienced it describe it as an unforgettable experience, in which one perceives a sort of liquid fire flowing up the sushumna, through the head and the top of the body.

CHAPTER 3: 7 NIGHTS OF TANTRA - GUIDE TO AWAKENING

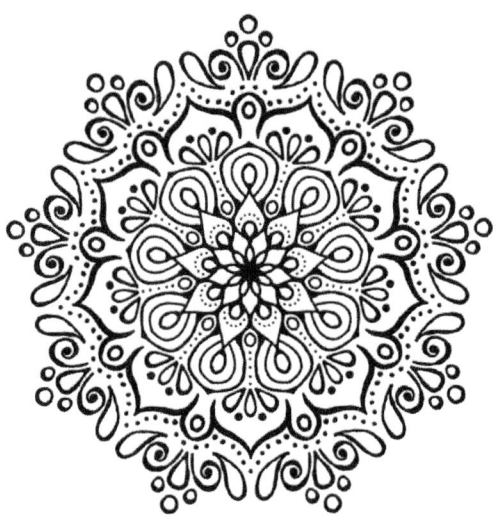

There is more and more talk of Tantra as a couple, of exercises, of making conscious love. For some people it is always a novelty, for others it is a source of income, and in any case something that should definitely be read and maybe practiced in couple because certainly the awareness in couple is essential for a lasting relationship. Lately I have also come across those who do courses with the secret techniques of the famous Seven Nights of Tantra. This makes me smile a lot, I remember that when I was teaching Yoga in my day these secret things were not. I wish you good reading.

The First of 7 Nights

Enter the rooms of the seven tantric nights.

Sitting at the table, drink a glass of wine, without touching the food and, after finishing it, kiss gently on the lips (just once).

The man stands up, in front of the woman and says: "I am ready".

The woman also stands up, stands in front of the man and starts to undress him, one garment after another, slowly, while he stands still with his arms left along his hips.

With each garment removed, the woman looks at the naked part of the man, without touching him, and recites the mantra of awareness ommm, ahdi, ommm.

When the man is completely naked, the woman also says: "I am ready" and the man slowly undresses her in the same way.

The man now begins the ritual of awareness as he is used to doing alone, but focusing on the image of the woman.

He touches her lips, nipples and pubis each time repeating the mantra of awareness ommm, ahdi, ommm.

With his eyes closed he focuses on the image of the woman, while she, with her eyes open, takes his hands and guides them, bringing them back to her lips, breasts and pubis.

The slowness of gestures is a source of pleasure and intimacy. At each contact is pronounced the mantra of awareness ommm, ahdi, ommm.

The woman, after being touched in this way, touches the man's lips with her thumb and index finger, then her nipple and then her pubis, taking the penis between her four fingers and gently squeezing the base. With her eyes closed, she visualizes his body and waits to be guided to touch it a second time.

Hug for a moment and separate. Sitting at the table, hold each other's hands in silence.

After a while you separate: everyone goes to a different room and repeats the rituals of control. Stop in time! At the threshold of orgasm stop, the climax of the pleasure will come later, sublimated.

Remaining in a different room, you also do the ritual of channeling.*

Then gather at the table, sitting on the pillows cross your hands repeating the mantra of awareness, ommm, ahdi, ommm. You will both be very excited, but avoid touching each other.

The 60-minute rule, which should not be violated at all, is strictly adhered to here. To distract yourself, eat and drink, talking quietly about what you want.

After spending a whole hour, go to the bedroom and do whatever you like. Devote yourself to sex in the way you prefer and enjoy unlimited sexual ecstasy. After both of you have reached orgasm, you can go to sleep, charged with sexual energy shaken, which will work for you while you rest and prepare for the second night.

*The channeling

It must be carried out after the masturbation and control phase.

In case you have anything you would like to solve, but don't know how, focus on one aspect of the problem and isolate it from everything else.

As you focus on your problem, repeat the mantra of channeling ahh, nahh, yahh, tawnnn, and think about channeling all the positive charges accumulated in pre orgasm to that particular situation.

Recite the mantra ahh, nahh, yahh, tawnnn, say something like: I will be able to eliminate that defect, or I will be able to overcome that obstacle, etc., and recite again the mantra ahh, nahh, yahh, tawnnn.

This operation must be done six times in a row. The sentence between the two mantras must be short and concise. The mantras must not contain reflections, but only the core of the problem. This will already help you. While you are busy doing something else, the accumulated energy will proceed directly to your problem, working for your well-being and harmony.

The Second of the 7 Nights

Sitting at the table as the night before, drink a glass of wine, thinking about the goal of the channeling.

It is the woman who begins: she stands up and says: "I am ready". The man, standing in front of her, begins to undress her, repeating the mantra of awareness ommm, ahdi, ommm.

When the man in turn says: "I am ready", the woman begins to undress him. Do not underestimate the importance of mantras and yantras, which have the delicate task of aligning your mind with the spirit and body.

Once naked both of you, embrace and kiss each other for a long time while standing, so that the only contact is between your naked bodies and your lips.

The second night now includes a bath, which you will proceed to separate rituals, like the night before.

You will find yourself sitting at the coffee table with your hands crossed.

In order to be able to control the excitement of the brushed orgasm, repeat the mantra of control pahhh, dahhh, o-mahmmm, and distract yourself by eating and drinking.

It is of paramount importance to respect the 60-minute rule.

After the 60-minute rule, move the cushions from the table and sit facing each other. The woman opens her legs by lifting her knees and the man crosses his legs to hers, placing his feet on her buttocks.

The hands should be placed on the partner's knees. This position is called "contemplative" and serves to establish mutual knowledge. The contact is very direct, even if the genitals are not touched.

Look into each other's eyes, then move your gaze to the breast, navel and pubis. With your eyes closed, focus your attention on the parts of the other, the woman imagine that the man penetrates her with his erect penis, ready to orgasm that floods her, and the man in turn imagine the vagina that, warm and open, welcomes him in pleasure.

Open your eyes at this point looking at your partner's genitals. Stand up and go into the bedroom. Take all the pleasure you can get, making love as you like. Let yourself go to the pleasure of the senses until you reach orgasm. Fall asleep in the awareness of the positive energies that will pass through you until the next night. Is beginning to please you, huh?

The Third of the 7 Nights

Always sitting at the table, drink a glass of wine and think, if you want to talk, about the goal of the channeling.

The man gets up and says the usual formula: "I'm ready".

He begins to undress slowly under the woman's gaze, until he is completely naked. He begins the ritual of awakening, while the woman, still and silent, looks at him until he is finished.

The woman then gets up, recites her "I am ready" and does the same thing under the gaze of the man. When she too has finished, hug and kiss each other while standing, so that the only contact is between the two bodies.

Then comes the moment of the bath, after which the man, lying down, will perform the ritual of awakening desire in the presence of the woman, sitting at the foot of the bed.

The woman carefully looks at the gestures that the man has made many times by himself, lying naked on the bed. When the man is finished, the woman will do the same thing under his gaze.

The ritual of control is then performed, but each one on his own. You absolutely must not have an orgasm, but only get very close to it and withdraw in time, otherwise the whole exercise becomes in vain.

After having also done the channeling separately, meet again at the table to eat, drink and chat, observing the rule of the 60 armed.

Then assume the contemplative position already experienced the previous night.

With eyes fixed on each other's genitals, the woman will lower herself to take the man's penis and testicles in her hands, following the movement of her index finger and thumb. The man focuses on the male yantric visualization and proceeds to muscle stimulation. The man contracts the muscles three times and the woman three times says, "I feel it.

Similarly, the man will lower himself towards the woman, inserting a finger into the vagina, but without stimulating other parts. The woman focuses on the female yantra visualization, and while she tightens the internal muscles three times, the man says "I feel it".

At this point you are free to go to the bedroom, where you will exchange all forms of pleasure in the way you like...until the next night.

The Fourth of the 7 Nights

As in the previous nights you will meet at the table, drinking a glass of wine together and talking openly about the objectives of the channeling. When the man says "I'm ready", he gets up and starts slowly undressing while the woman looks at him. The woman, too, after saying "I am ready", undresses.

Both naked, hug and kiss each other and go to the bathroom.

Go back to the coffee table and, sitting on the pillows, assume the position of contemplation: the woman takes the penis in her hands while the man commands the contraction three times, then the man puts a finger in the vagina, while she three times tightens the muscles.

To this you will do something you have probably never done before.

On the fourth night of tantra, the man and woman perform the entire ritual of control under the eyes of their partner, i.e. a full-fledged masturbation, which stops at the threshold of orgasm.

While the man masturbates the woman sitting at the foot of the bed in silence, without ever touching him or herself. The man will then do the same thing. This practice allows a new confidence, which is achieved only through a gradual overcoming of the barriers between man and woman. Watch carefully every little movement of the other, so that you can learn the best way to touch him/her.

Sit down at the table and, observing the 60-minute rule, eat and drink, chatting. When you have finished, you can hold hands and go to the bedroom, where you will make love in the way you prefer, without inhibitions and in full of the new confidence reached.

In view of the fifth night, rest well, while the energies released in intercourse will work to improve your life during sleep.

The Fifth of the 7 Nights

Sitting at the table drink a glass of wine and talk about the goal you want to achieve. The woman starts by saying "I'm ready" and slowly undressing. In turn the man says "I'm ready" and undresses.

Completely naked, hug and kiss each other, and go to the bathroom.

Move the cushions from the table and sit down in the position of contemplation. Just like the night before, the man will feel the muscular stimulus of the woman and vice versa. Then go together into the bedroom, where the woman will lie down with her legs open and her feet painte that match.

It will be the man this time, sitting next to the woman, who will start to touch her: first the lips, then the breasts and then the pubis.

As he did with himself, the man touches the woman only as indicated, as he is accustomed to doing during the ritual of control.

The gestures must be slow and decisive. Touch her lips with your fingers, with your palms open, take her breasts in your hand, gently squeezing the top and gently stimulate her nipple.

Put your hands down on her belly, and place them on hers, crossed under the navel. Stop a little and then go down to the pubis. With your thumbs open your lips and touch the clitoris making a light rotating movement.

He says: "I feel it", and she answers "I feel it" only when the man touches her in the best way. To do this she can lead his fingers to the exact point of pleasure.

The man must understand well what are the points on which to apply the right pressure, grasping the reactions of the partner.

Attention: the man is performing the ritual of control on the woman's body. This means that both of you absolutely must not let go. Control is the foundation of tantra and without it everything loses sense and effectiveness. If the difficulty is too high, interrupt.

The woman then, sitting at the edge of the bed, will touch the man, taking care not to make him come. She will have to pay particular attention because he will be very excited. After touching his lips and nipples, she puts her hands on his belly and then goes down to his pubis. Taking his penis in her hands, she makes the gestures that she saw him make the night before. A moment before coming, the man grabs the woman's arm, so that she stops the contact immediately. The moment requires silence, respect and intimacy.

Go to the table and distract yourself by eating and drinking. After an hour, go to the bedroom and exchange pleasure without limits, no longer worrying about control.

The orgasm you will have will be the strongest you have ever experienced.

The Sixth of the 7 Nights

You find yourself sitting at the table, drinking a glass of wine. The bathroom, the contemplative position, the exercise of contractions and the embrace.

The woman lies on the bed and says "I am ready". The man, sitting next to her, dedicates himself to her pleasure. With the tip of his index finger he touches her lips, puts his palms on her face and with his tongue follows the contours of her lips. He kisses her passionately, while she remains passive, focused on her feelings.

He goes down to her breasts, taking one nipple at a time between his fingers. He squeezes it a little between his fingers and massages the entire breast. Then she takes the nipple between her lips and sucks it lightly, first one and then the other. She descends towards the pubis, while the woman always remains with her hands intertwined on the abdomen.

The man opens the woman's lips with his thumbs and touches the clitoris with the tip of his index finger. He then places his hands on the vagina for a few seconds and starts again.

Open your lips again and go down to the perineum with your fingertips, exerting gentle pressure, go down again until you touch the rectum and press down lightly. Place your hands on her vagina and stay still for a few seconds.

Man's oral sex on woman

Open your lips with your fingers and lean towards her sex, take one in your mouth and suck it gently. Then do the same with the other. Stick your tongue into her vagina and move it from top to bottom. Continue licking up towards the clitoris and suck it gently.

Every reaction of the woman is a precious indication for the man, who chooses from time to time how to proceed, between one intensity and another. The moment the woman is about to come, she warns her partner by grabbing him, so that he immediately stops. You absolutely must not reach orgasm, it will be afterwards. Here the woman visualizes and channels.

Then comes the turn of man's pleasure.

If the man is very excited, it is good to wait a moment before starting. In any case, the woman will wait for the phrase: "I am ready".

Follow the profile of your partner's lips with the tip of your index finger. Place the palms of your hands on his face and touch his lips with your tongue. Kiss him passionately, while he remains passive. Place your hands on his breasts, take a nipple between your fingers and gently stimulate it. Bring your mouth to the nipple and suck it, first one and then the other.

With your hands down on his hands, cross his abdomen. Go down again taking the base of the penis between two fingers. The penis must be touched by running it all the way from the glans to under the scrotum and perineum, then up again to the top. When you reach the top, squeeze the glans with two fingers, so that it slightly decreases in size (air escapes). Then touch the perineum and rectum, exerting nothing more than a slight pressure.

Leave your hands at the edges of the genitals for a moment, then return to the base of the penis in its deepest part. Hold it at the base with just two fingers, while the rest of your hand holds his testicles.

The oral sex of the woman on the man

The penis is erect and the glans presses on the belly. Without moving your hands, press with your mouth on the base of the penis, and go up to the glans, covering your teeth with your lips. At the top, move the penis so that it is perpendicular to your body. In this position uncover the glans and suck it, moving your tongue in a circular motion.

With the right hand hold the base, while with the other hand the testicles, making a slight pressure on the perineum and rectum. Suck the glans by moving your head up and down to cover as much of the penis as possible. The movements should be calibrated according to your partner's reactions. When he signals you to stop, detach immediately.

The man should now concentrate and control his impulses effectively, using visualization and channeling techniques.

In the next hour, eat, talk, distract yourself and then go back to bed, where at this point the pleasure you will feel is unimaginable if you do not experience it...

The Seventh and Last Night of Tantric Sex

Drinking a glass of wine sitting at the table, talk about the personal goal to be achieved through the channeling. Strip each other and go to the bathroom. Back at the table, assume the contemplative position, including muscle contractions.

Go together to the bedroom. The woman lies down with her legs apart, assuming the usual position and the man touches her lips, breast and pubis.

In this circumstance you need a lot of attention from both of them.

At every gesture of the man, the woman must openly say everything she feels and feels, without leaving anything out. She must try to be very precise and clear, indicating which are the gestures and points that give her the most pleasure.

After a few minutes the man lies down in place of the woman. While she touches his face he expresses his feelings, after she kisses him, he tells her what he felt. She massages his breasts and touches his nipples, and he describes everything as she continues.

When you have an erection in your hands, put yourself on top of him and, widening your lips, slide it inside of you, very slowly. The formulas of the I am ready must precede this operation, and mantras and yantras accompany the whole session.

As he penetrates you, tighten your muscles and do the yanthra visualization, the man in turn does the same. You both say, "I feel it. When you have done this, lie next to each other for a few minutes and then begin to touch each other, making love as you like.

CHAPTER 4: TIPS TO ENHANCE YOUR INTERCOURSE

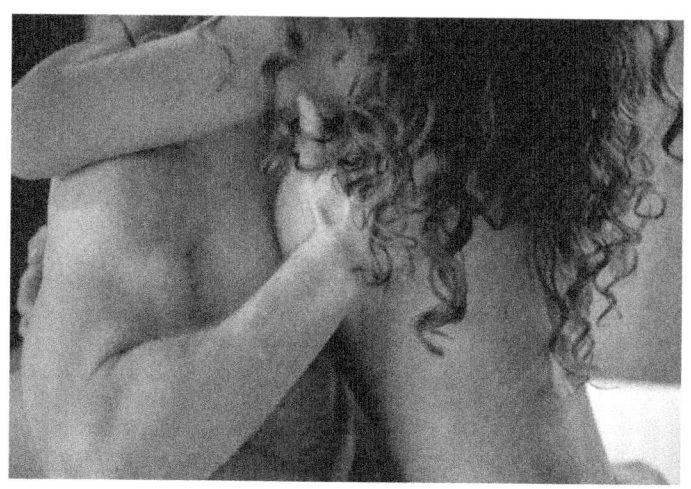

Tantric Exercises

Having strong sexual muscles is the basis to become a tantric lover, otherwise it is impossible to think to control them and successfully practice Tantra.

There is a specific group of muscles that surrounds the sexual organs, which is extremely important for the general health and functioning of the latter. The correct name for these muscles is pubo-coccygeal or "PC muscle", as we usually prefer to call them. We refer to this group of muscles as one muscle because it functions as a unit during sexual activity, but it can actually be divided into three areas:

- the area around the anus;

- the area of the perineum, between the anus and sex;

- the area around the sex.

A strong and trained "PC muscle" is the key to good sexuality for both men and women.

Contractions of the PC muscle

One of the best ways to train the PC muscle is to do contractions. When you start doing contractions, most likely you will not be able to split the PC muscle into its 3 parts, but you will contract the whole area. Don't worry, it's normal. With time and effort you will be able to feel them, and train them separately. Below we propose a very effective training, which includes 2 types of contractions.

Short contractions

Quickly contract and relax the PC muscle (or part of it) by holding the contraction for 1 second and releasing for 1 second. 10 consecutive sequences are performed for each sequence; five sequences are done for each training session that will be done once a day.

Long contractions

Contract and relax the PC muscles by holding the contraction for 30 seconds and releasing for 2 seconds. 3 consecutive contractions are performed for each sequence. Five sequences are done for each session which will be done once a day.

Karezza

Karezza is a very important technique that helps men and women to perceive and control sexual energies; it is said that the name comes from the Italian word "Carezza", but not all historians agree. It is based on the fact that the man penetrates the woman, and then the beloved ones remain embraced completely immobile; no movement is allowed. When the man loses his erection, he comes out of the penetration. The lovers get excited again, and the technique begins again.

Let's see the advantages:

- very useful for men who want to learn sexual continence
- It helps a lot the harmonization of the couple, it is therefore ideal to practice it in times of tension and difficulty.
- he helps to become more sensitive to each other and energies, coming to grasp even small nuances.

- shows how beautiful and deep can be even the simple contact of the sexual organs, without any need for the chase to orgasm and ejaculation

Erotic massage

We all remember with great pleasure when we were taken in our arms, touched and pampered by our parents. Every caress to our body, was really a caress to our heart. Massage is a very important part in the relationship of a couple; you should massage often. It is a deep way to know our body and that of the loved one. But above all, it is a way of awakening the body; in fact, the more it is massaged, the more sensitive it becomes and opens up to pleasure.

It is The Tantric massage follows some principles:

1. Concentration

While I massage I am 100% focused on what I am doing, I don't think about the movements I will make afterwards, or the areas I will massage, I don't set goals,

I don't look for results, I don't have expectations, I let emotions and sensations flow, and I abandon myself in the present moment.

2. Relaxation

There is nothing worse than a person who is not relaxed when massaging; the partner feels it immediately. One of the best ways to relax is to calm your breathing, which must be slow and deep, and center ourselves.

● **Let's follow the technique, but also the heart**

Massage is a real art; learning to massage in this way, with an open heart, and with consciousness and attention, we will develop a strong intuition. This will allow us to understand what our partner likes or dislikes, and to modify the sequences during the massage. It may be that on that day he prefers to be massaged longer on his legs, because he has spent a lot of time on his feet, or on his back, because he is tense.

- **Fluidity**

The massage is like a dance, it is not made of a series of separate movements, but they are all connectedEach gesture serves to perfect the previous one, and to prepare the next one.The flow is continuous, there are no interruptions.

- **Request feedback to our loved one**

Especially at the first massages, let's not be ashamed to ask what he likes, and which areas he prefers to be massaged. This will help us a lot to turn a simple massage into an ecstatic experience for our partner. When we already know our partner, then it is better to remain silent. There are of course different types of tantric massage sequences, which we teach in our courses.

Tantric Techniques To Rebalance Energies

Tantric meditation: to rebalance energies (individual or in pairs). Lie on your back and start breathing until the flow becomes slow and deep. When you reach this moment imagine that, together with the inhalation, from the top of your head a golden light enters inside you and comes out of your toes. As you exhale you will see a black light coming out from the top of your head. To practice every evening for about twenty minutes.

Bioenergetic meditation: to enter the present (in pairs). Lie on your back and concentrate on your breathing. Feel the flow of air at each inhalation and exhalation, listen to the sensations in your chest as your muscles release to let air into your lungs and, as they contract, to let it out. Extend awareness to the whole body and emotions in the present moment. Open your eyes by holding your breathing and sending your inner power and presence to the outside world that you will in turn receive within you. Perform in the evening to free yourself from thoughts.

Bioenergetic Breathing: to get rid of blocks (in pairs). Lie on your back, relax and start breathing slowly. Focus on the flow of your breath and try to figure out whether you are breathing with your chest or abdomen. Then start breathing into your chest, until you feel your heart open and create a comfortable position. Then move on to the stomach, belly (two fingers below the navel), genitals and perineum. Pay attention to the breathing condition in the various areas: if you feel a blockage, help yourself with a local massage by keeping your legs bent.

Tantric Sexual intercourse: Useful Tips

For the elasticity of the pelvis (for her): lie on your back, bend your legs and spread them slightly. Start breathing slowly focusing on the breath. Keep the contact of the back with the mattress or the ground and push the pelvis back and forth (inhaling and exhaling) with a rhythmic and harmonic movement. Make no effort but achieve pleasure for ten, fifteen minutes.

To enter the other: sit comfortably, in an upright position. Close your eyes focusing on the sensations that your body communicates to you. Open your eyes, observe yourself and immerse yourself in the gaze of the other by tuning your thoughts with the same rhythm. Do not worry if you burst into tears or if you feel like laughing. Express yourself freely for about a quarter of an hour, then place your hands on your chest and bow your head with a bow of greeting.

During intercourse: lie on him or by his side and relax. Begin to breathe slowly tuning the rhythm of inhalation and exhalation to each other. Feel all the sensations. Do not rush and stop every now and then: hurried breathing accelerates the ejaculation, deep breathing helps to prolong the intercourse. If you both focus your attention on breathing, you will automatically bring it to the heart region as well. The shifting of energy from the genitals to the heart amplifies and prolongs the dimension of the sexual act. Do not hold your breath while waiting for orgasm, but relax your breathing in a global expansion of energy. Don't lose heart if things don't work right away: you are overloaded with sedimented patterns that you need to get rid of and this cannot happen quickly!

For the afterwards: avoid running to the bathroom to wash or turning on your side to sleep. Let yourself fall as if you were dead, then hold your hands, breathe together and look into each other's eyes trying to convey to each other all the emotions you felt. If you spontaneously joke, laugh and chat. Try to observe your breathing: if the solar plexus has widened, it is the heart that has expanded and will give you a sense of peace and happiness.

Some advice...

- First of all, learn to love yourself.

- Do not be in a hurry.

- Do not think about orgasm.

- Let yourself go completely without fear.

- Focus on your feelings.

- Learn to breathe correctly.

- Eliminate thoughts and immerse yourself in the present moment.

- Accept your partner for who he is and trust him.

- Be aware of your body and the sexual act.

- If there is a problem with premature ejaculation, go to the pre-ejaculation stage and, with finger pressure at the base of the glans, block the outflow (Taoist advice and modern sexology).

- Do not always use the same positions in the intercourse (she below and he above is the worst).

- Remember that the contemporary orgasm is more a myth than a reality.

- Get out of the schemes that have been imposed on you in order to reach the mystical orgasm.

The Way Of Tao And The Way Of Tantra

The Tao is a form of wisdom from thousands of years ago. No one knows exactly when it was born. One has to wait until the 4th century B.C. to find its fundamental precepts expressed in a book, the Tao Tê Ching by Lao Tzu. The Tao is the infinite force of nature, its philosophy is to endure and to succeed in this it is necessary to be relaxed and natural. The first Chinese doctors started writing about love and sex two thousand years ago. They were Taoists and for them making love was part of the natural order of things. Sex was not only enjoyed and savored, but considered a healthy and life-extending activity. Taoist doctrine encourages men to develop control of ejaculation and teaches that orgasm and ejaculation are not the same thing: having less ejaculation does not mean being sexually inadequate or experiencing less sexual pleasure but, on the contrary, it means increasing mental lucidity, body strength and sharpening of sight and hearing. Instead of an explosion of tension, it causes a pleasure of peace, a sensual, lasting and satisfying union with something greater than ourselves, which blends yin and yiang (feminine and masculine) into harmony.

Tantra, on the other hand, originates in India. Tantric arts are often confused with Taoism but, although Tantrism may have been influenced or even originated from Tao, its various schools have developed a different philosophy, much more linked to rituality. The Tantra, as an esoteric/philosophical body, was systematized around the fourth century BC but its origins, much older, are not known. The tantric texts were written in Sanskrit and spoke of sexual understanding as a moment of mutual knowledge between two people.

In the tantric type of union in fact the man and the woman join together aware that they are the two aspects (male and female) of the divinity. This is why tantra teaches the integration of body, mind and spirit in order to develop the most sublime forms of pleasure. Among the various tantric practices, great importance is given to relaxation and touching each other, so as to allow the detachment of the mind from everyday life to go towards total satisfaction. Even haste is not recommended in a lasting and satisfying sexual relationship, because it distracts us from all the components as well as speeding up the conclusion without considering the pleasure and mutual communication that precedes it.

How To Help Reaching Orgasm

Chromotherapy

An intense light in shades ranging from green to blue applied to the solar plexus, lumbar region, forehead and temples slows down a male performance too fast. To help her achieve orgasm, blue light should be applied on the coccyx, while orange is indicated on the ovaries and the center of the forehead. If you do not have the right instrument for color therapy, you can opt for a light of the desired heat, or apply on the affected parts of the fabric in the chosen shade. In the morning, fill a colored glass bottle with water (blue or reddish/orange, depending on the problem), expose it to the sun all day and drink its contents in the evening.

Floritherapy

The Sticky Monkeyflower is a Californian flower that helps to overcome fear of intimacy, to shed light on confusions related to sexuality and to integrate life force and sexuality. The Manzanita is another Californian flower, its main function is to lead us to love and care for our body. Clematis, in Bach flowers, is the remedy for those who are distracted, evade the fantasy and can not live the here and now. Cherry Plum is a Bach flower suitable for those who are afraid of losing control and instead helps to have confidence in life and let go without fearing the judgments of others. Fuchsia is a Californian remedy for those who are afraid of strong emotions and therefore tend to control them mentally, but also for those who repress them.

Homeopathy

For him: Damiana Compositum, Selenium 9ch (three granules three times a day for twenty days), Phosphoricum acidum 9ch (three granules three times a day for a week).

For her: Onosmodium 9ch (to revitalize the absent desire), Eleutherococcus senticosus in mother tincture (thirty drops once a day).

Aromatherapy

Recommended essences to be placed in the aroma lamp: fill the tray and add five to fifteen drops of essential oils, light the candle under the container and the effluent will expand into the room. The essences with sensual effect are: ylang-ylang, sandalwood, neroli, rose, cedar, patchouli. You can also make combinations (two drops of ylang-ylang and five of sandalwood, or two drops of neroli, five of sandalwood, two of cedar and three of rose). For a sensual bath, mix ten drops of sandalwood, three drops of ylang-ylang with three tablespoons of honey and two of cream.

CONCLUSION

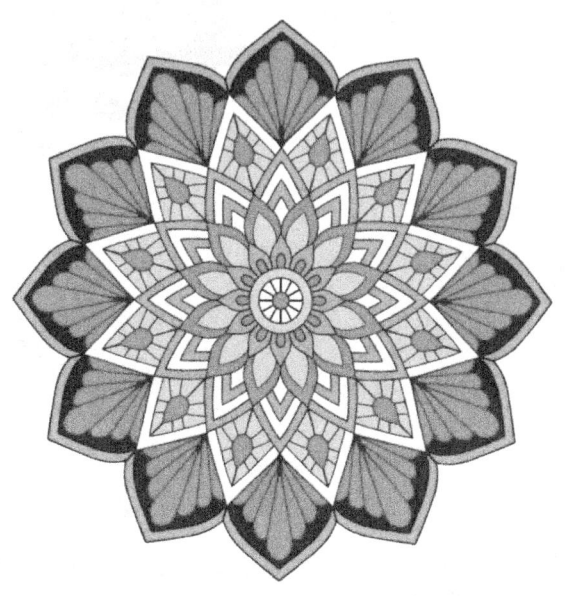

This book has come to the conclusion, we have learned how Tantric sex is an entirely "oriental" method of making love.

The well-known singer Sting, for example, is a big supporter of it. It is said, in fact, that the well-known singer is able to make love with his wife Trudy for about seven hours in a row, without ever getting tired. But how is this possible? It is, precisely, through tantric sex. In essence, it is a very different way of having sex. It is something that approaches Eastern disciplines, such as yoga for example.

It allows to rekindle the flame of passion, but not only.

Tantric is a type of sex that is performed very calmly. It goes without saying that in it there is no performance anxiety, premature ejaculation and the like. It is not something aimed at orgasm, contrary to what you might think and unlike sex to which we Westerners are accustomed. It is, in essence, something higher, purely mental, which is about spiritual communion.

It is a real life experience, which is worth trying.

Tantric sex is certainly not to be confused with the Kamasutra. The latter, in fact, concerns sexual positions. It is something purely different, even if it is also part of the Eastern discipline. There are, in any case, perfect positions for this type of sex, in this type of sexual intercourse, it is the woman who has an active approach. She transfers her cold energy to the man, who in turn transforms it into hot energy. In addition, it is essential to look into each other's eyes, creating a deep connection. Now it's to experience everything by yourself...I hope you enjoyed this book, have fun!

Printed in Great Britain
by Amazon

53252744R00068